THE
LITTLE
BOOK
OF
Sex Secrets

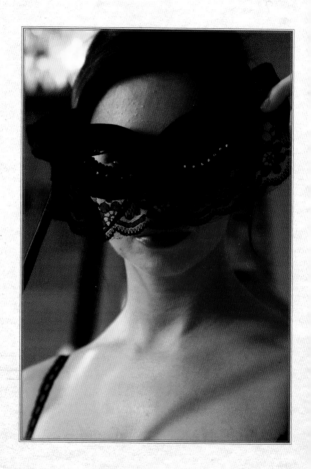

THE
LITTLE
BOOK
OF

Sex Secrets

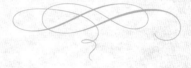

NICOLE
BAILEY

RED-HOT CONFESSIONS, FANTASIES,
TECHNIQUES & DISCOVERIES

DUNCAN BAIRD PUBLISHERS
LONDON

The Little Book of Sex Secrets

NICOLE BAILEY

This edition first published in the United Kingdom and Ireland in 2013 by
Duncan Baird Publishers Ltd, Sixth Floor, Castle House, 75–76 Wells Street
London W1T 3QH

Conceived, created and designed by Duncan Baird Publishers

Managing Editor: Grace Cheetham
Editors: Dawn Bates and Ingrid Court-Jones
Managing Designer: Manisha Patel
Art Direction and Design: Sailesh Patel
Commissioned Photography: John Davis

British Library Cataloguing-in-Publication Data:
A CIP record for this book is available from the British Library

ISBN: 978-1-84899-066-1
10 9 8 7 6 5 4 3 2 1

Typeset in MrsEaves & Bickham Script Pro
Colour reproduction by Scanhouse, Malaysia
Printed in Thailand by Imago

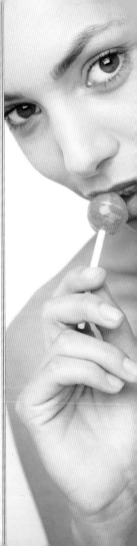

Contents

Introduction

Whenever I get together with my female friends, quite often the conversation slowly but surely turns to sex. We share experiences from the past and present, as well as fantasies about the future. I love these conversations with other women. As well as being fun, they're also liberating, enlightening and informative – I've learnt so much from them. This was one of my main inspirations for writing *The Little Book of Sex Secrets*: to share my own experiences and those of other women. After all there's something very valuable about being given a sex tip that's already been tried and tested.

BE A CONFIDENT SEDUCTRESS

As well as tips on how to flirt, talk dirty and take your clothes off, I've included dozens of secrets to build your sexual confidence. My hope is that you'll find and enjoy your inner seductress. Sometimes seduction can be subtle: looks, touches, gestures and a flirtatious undercurrent that runs through your conversations. Other times it's big and brazen, like when you lure him into the bedroom and perform a mesmerizing striptease to music. Seduction techniques might seem as though they're all for his pleasure, but you'll find them just as thrilling as he does.

HAVE STIMULATING FOREPLAY

I've included my favourite foreplay techniques, from slow and sensual massage to red-hot oral sex techniques. And, because women tell me how much they appreciate the right kind of arousal, I've shared the secrets of getting him to touch you the way you want.

TREAT SEX AS AN ADVENTURE

I love being playful and daring in bed. I've included my favourite games and naughty activities, plus those of other women. For example, how to play sex dares, make an erotic film or arouse each other with sexy power games. And if you have an "I-can't-do-that" moment, I hope that the sexual confessions and anecdotes will inspire you to leave your comfort zone. It's worth it!

Nicole Bailey

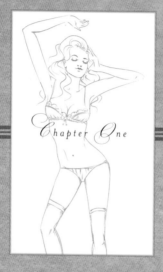

Chapter One

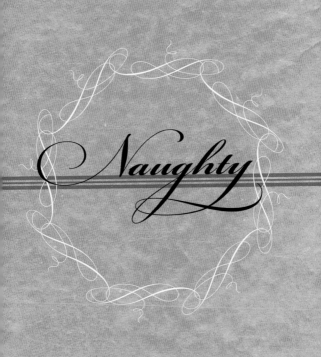

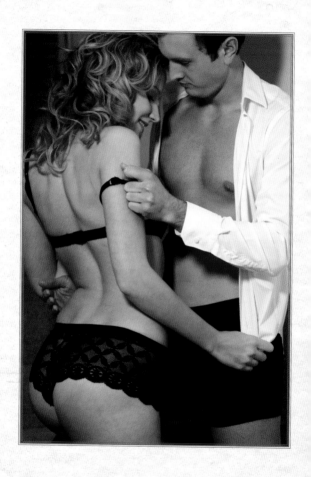

Naughty

The Art of Arousal

What better place to start than with foreplay – being fully aroused is at the heart of sexual satisfaction. My top tip is that whatever your favourite type of foreplay, do it wholeheartedly. My favourite is slow and exploratory kissing that builds to a passionate tongue-twining crescendo.

GET INTO THE GROOVE

Good foreplay is like good dancing, so find a natural rhythm and don't worry about the moves. Forget scripted ideas of what foreplay "should" be and, remember, foreplay doesn't have to lead to sex – it can be the main event. My female friends have told me their top foreplay moments:

"I loved it when he sucked my fingers as he caressed me."

"He pushed my legs apart and just breathed hotly on my clitoris. Then he started teasing me with little cat licks."

"In the shower – he wrapped his arms around me from behind and started playing with my nipples. Then I turned round and went down on him."

USE MIRRORING

If he takes a sip of his drink, take one, too. If he changes position, change yours to match. Unconsciously, he'll be flattered that you're so highly in tune with him. In my experience, it's good to keep your moves subtle. Go for reflection rather than obvious mimicry of his gestures and body language.

LAVISH HIM WITH COMPLIMENTS

Gaze directly at your partner and tell him how funny, intelligent, sexy or loveable he is. Most importantly, make sure you mean it.

TEASE HIM

Try playfully withholding sex. It'll make him feel he's got to seduce, entice and woo you. I try never to be a sure thing (even if I am!).

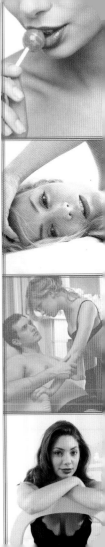

MAKE IT PUBLIC

Flirt outrageously with your man in front of his friends. I've found that my lover adores the flattery when his friends can see I've only got eyes for him.

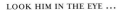

LOOK HIM IN THE EYE ...

and hold his gaze. Don't speak. Even if you know each other inside out, prolonged eye contact feels unsettling and exciting. Gaze appreciatively at his lips, too (I always imagine giving my lover a hot, sexy kiss at this point).

BE NAUGHTY

Use symbolic gestures: purse your lips around a straw as you're drinking or suck a lollipop and gaze up at him as you do so. Briefly lick your lips or twine your hair in your fingers.

15

Talk Dirty

My first boyfriend converted me to the joys of talking dirty. I was feeling sleepy, but my tiredness vanished as he whispered in my ear, "Open your legs, I want to lick you." The sex that followed was hot! Once I experienced the naughty power of words, I suddenly got it: sex felt more adult, X-rated and exciting.

THE POWER OF WORDS

- You can change your entire sexual persona instantly. There's no faster way to go from good girl to wicked girl.
- You've got a readily available sex tool at your disposal — any time, any place. No one else need know.
- If your lover's erection is flagging, dirty talk can send blood rushing straight to where it's needed.
- If you're apart, you can have amazing phone sex.
- If you usually have sweet, lovey-dovey sex, dirty talk can charge up your sex life and make you see each other in a completely different — and more exciting — light.

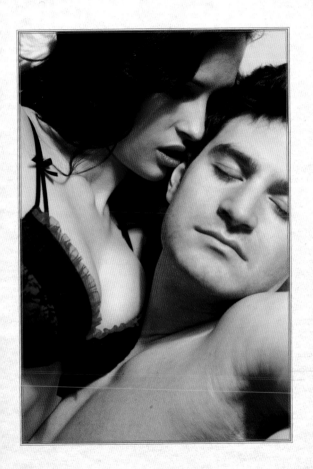

Naughty

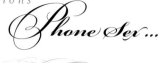
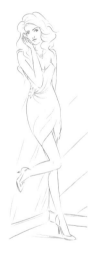

MY LOVER WAS LATE TO MEET ME FOR DINNER LAST WEEK. Rather than leaving me unoccupied in the restaurant, he called my mobile and described in detail all the wicked things he planned to do to me later on. For 20 minutes I blushed and said "uh huh" and "oh, really?" as the restaurant filled up with prim-looking diners. Several times I said "I have to go now", but he wouldn't let me hang up. In fact any sign of embarrassment just spurred him on to new heights of depravity. I secretly loved it. It reminded me what a titillating tool the phone is. Here are some confessions from other phone sex fans:

"My boyfriend has a deep, gravelly voice that's perfect for phone sex — it's aroused me since the day we met. It's strange to say, but I almost enjoy sex on the phone as much as sex in the flesh. I dress in my sexiest underwear and stockings, and then lie on top of the bed caressing myself while I wait for him to call (we agree a time in advance to get the full thrill of anticipation). I love the moment when the phone rings — I still get butterflies in my stomach. And when I pick up he never bothers with saying hello — he just says my name softly. I've never told him how aroused I get by this."

"My partner and I once decided to phone a sex phone line out of sheer curiosity. It was more funny than erotic — neither of us could take the breathy panting seriously. But it did have an amazingly sexy side-effect, freeing us of our own inhibitions. Now phone sex is a really fast way for both of us to have an orgasm when we're apart. It brings out our filthiest sides."

BE SEXY OUTSIDE THE BEDROOM

Let your lover know you think he's hot all the time, both in bed and out. Trail your fingers across his buttocks; gently caress his chest and belly; nuzzle his neck; nibble ears.

REMEMBER THE FIRST TIME

Describe to him the time you first met/ kissed/made love. Tell him in graphic detail all the things you fancied about him – and still do.

MAKE MORNINGS SEXY

If sex was fantastic last night, whisper in his ear when he wakes up. For example, "I loved what you did to me last night, especially the way you dominated me." Then let your hands drift down to discover his morning erection.

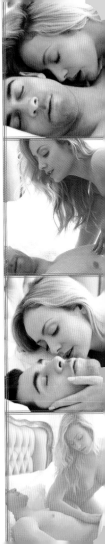

BE PLAYFUL

When you go for dinner with friends,
agree a "trigger" word in advance,
such as "delicious", "taste", "sauce".
When someone says the word, you
must caress each other under the
table, or kiss.

DO IT ANYWAY

There will always be times when you're
tired and not in the mood – but get
passionate anyway. I guarantee that
after five minutes of heavy smooching,
your body will catch up.

PLAY THE COMPLIMENT GAME

You give him a compliment and
he returns it – now just keep going.
Sex is great when you're both high
on intense mutual admiration.

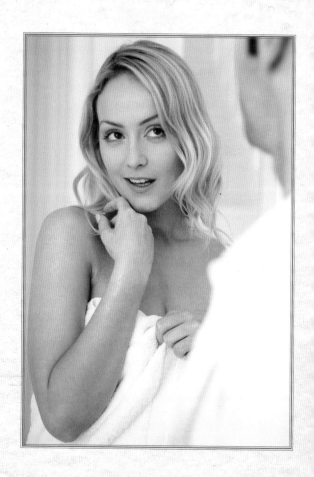

Naughty

Be Adventurous

Treat sex as an opportunity to be creative. Instead of following a formula of, say, stilettos, silk knickers and satin sheets, try talking dirty, reading erotica or tantalizing him with slow, sensual foreplay.

SET THE MOOD TO HOT

Close your eyes and imagine the scene: your lover is on his way over and the only thought on your mind is that first kiss. It may be tempting to pounce on him as soon he arrives, but instead try this …

Take a shower and greet him wearing only a towel. Kiss, then leave him to simmer while you change into something provocative. Flirt, turning up the heat a degree at a time: move a little closer, hold his gaze and show off your sexiest assets. When he touches you, respond with slow sensuality. Pull back after each kiss, look into his eyes and tell him how good he tastes. Give him cooling-off time by popping to the bathroom. Prolong the anticipation …

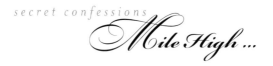

Mile High ...

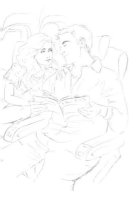

ONE OF MY FAVOURITE SEXUAL EXPERIENCES took place on a New York to London flight. My boyfriend fell asleep just after take-off — a fact that alarmed me because I'm terrified of flying. The flight turned out to be really turbulent, and when my boyfriend woke up, I was tired, edgy and anxious. And we were beginning the descent — my least favourite part of the flight. "I've got something for your nerves," he said sleepily. I looked at him doubtfully. He handed me a slim package loosely wrapped in black tissue paper and lace. I slid the lace off and peeked inside — it was a book. On the cover a woman was lying naked with her legs apart and her head thrown back in rapture. The title was something along the lines of *Kinky Stories for Girls*.

I thrust the book back in the paper, worried someone would see it. My boyfriend, delighting in my embarrassment, slid it inside a magazine, then opened it at a page he'd bookmarked. He leant close so his lips were nearly touching my ear. "I'm going to read you a story," he whispered in his husky, just-woken-up voice. Then he whispered an incredibly explicit story in my ear. Fittingly, it was about a couple having sex in a plane toilet. As he whispered expletives I could feel my anxiety disappearing and arousal taking its place. When he got to the climactic ending of the story, I was completely turned on. I was desperate for us to be off the plane so that I could kiss and touch him. As we were coming in to land, he got a flimsy plane blanket, pulled it over our laps and leant in to caress me …

INDULGE

Treat yourself to a sex toy, a slinky dress, a pampering session or lovely lingerie (even when no one will see it).

DISCOVER YOUR "HOT TIMES"

Lots of women have told me that they feel sexy around mid-cycle (when they ovulate). I've noticed it, too. Keep a diary of your cycle, and then tie in a date with your lover.

KNOW YOUR SEXUAL SELF

Know what makes you climax (and what doesn't); know where your G-spot is (see page 133); know what turns you on. Don't wait for your lover to unlock your sexuality – make sure you get there first.

USE THE POWER OF YOUR IMAGINATION

Close your eyes and picture yourself as a sexy goddess – someone who's comfortable in her own skin; who adores giving and receiving pleasure; and who loves to touch, tease, flirt and dance. Be that person in bed tonight.

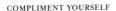

COMPLIMENT YOURSELF

Look in the mirror and say "I've got great breasts"/"I'm gorgeous"/"I love my hair"/"My curves are sexy". Keep a "mental bank" of the compliments people pay you.

SHOW OFF YOUR SEXINESS

Dress to show off your assets; connect with people through eye contact; be tactile; laugh and smile; try to be uninhibited and proud of your body when you're naked.

STOP WISHING, START ACTING

Wish you were slimmer/younger/prettier? Make a list of the things you'd do if you could attain your ideal appearance. Now do them anyway.

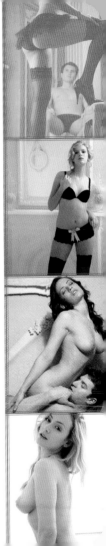

27

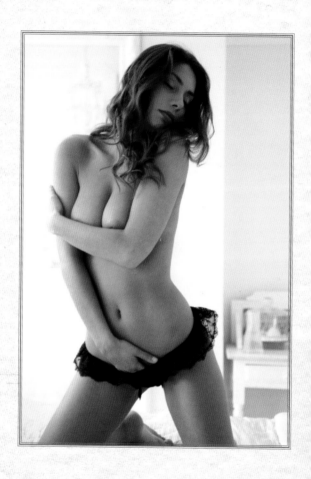

Naughty

Orgasms – Yours and His

My orgasms come in all shapes and sizes.
Sometimes they're frequent; sometimes they're elusive.
Sometimes they're slight and sometimes they send me
flying. But the more I understand how orgasms work,
the more control I seem to have over them.

SENSATIONAL SENSATIONS

I've discovered orgasms can come in a variety of ways. In fact,
orgasms don't even have to involve contact with the genitals.

Back in the 1970s researchers collected students'
descriptions of their orgasms. Any references to penises,
vaginas and clitorises were removed, and the descriptions
were then presented to a group of judges. The result? The
judges couldn't tell the difference between the account of a
male and a female orgasm. For fun, ask your lover to describe
his orgasms – and describe yours. You may end up tearing
each other's clothes off. Here's how some friends of mine
described their orgasms:

"A sudden rush – euphoria followed by deep relaxation."

"Convulsions all over my body that feel fantastic."

"An exciting build up of tension, then sudden, fast relief."

"A deep craving that I can't ignore, then deep satisfaction."

"A wave that comes and engulfs me. Time stops."

HIS ORGASM – HOW TO KNOW IT'S COMING

Here's what you need to know about how he climaxes:

- Unlike women, men reach a "point of no return" – this happens a few seconds before he actually ejaculates. Once he's got to this stage, it's impossible to prevent orgasm and ejaculation (even if you withdraw all stimulation from his penis). Signs that he's reaching the point of no return are: his testicles are drawn up tightly to his body; his glans has deepened in colour; his body is tense, stiff or jerky; he's moaning uncontrollably.

- If he's got a solid erection and droplets of pre-ejaculate on the tip of his glans, he's extremely aroused – if he's getting plenty of rhythmic stimulation on his shaft, the point of no return probably won't be far off.

Ask him to go for several days without ejaculating (whether by masturbation or intercourse). His next orgasm will be much more powerful.

YOUR ORGASM — THE BEST ROUTE

*T*ry these suggestions to climax during intercourse:

- Wait until you're super-excited before you have sex.
- Add frills! Depending on the sex position you're in, add masturbation or slip a vibrating toy between your bodies.
- Enjoy a hand-, toy- or tongue-delivered orgasm before or after sex.
- Find out if there are any sex positions that tip you over the edge. Woman-on-top positions can help because they put you in control and you can bump and grind against his pubic bone.
- Minimize distractions — orgasms are notoriously difficult to come by if you're preoccupied or stressed. Keep your mind busy by moaning your lover's name, gasping with pleasure or talking dirty.
- The more you hope to climax, the more elusive orgasm can become. Try reverse psychology: tell yourself you won't have an orgasm. If you don't, that's fine. If you do, it'll be relaxed and enjoyable.

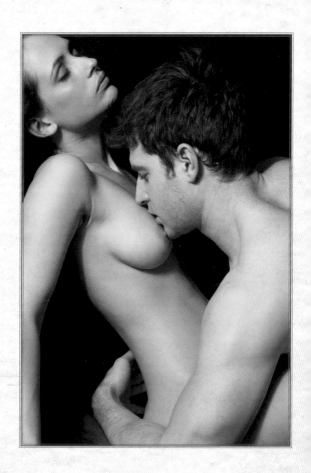

Naughty

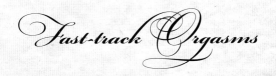

Fast-track Orgasms

Although long, lingering sex sessions are fantastic,
I don't always have time for them. That's why it's good
to know some quick routes to orgasm. The trick is to
do something genuinely surprising — and something
extremely sexy.

TAKE CONTROL

· Swallow your inhibitions and masturbate in front of him.

· Join him in the shower. He'll love your impulsiveness.

· Men like genital close ups — he'll love it if you greet him in
bed with your legs apart. Or adopt a sex position you want
to try — before he enters the bedroom.

· If you tend to initiate sex, withdraw completely. When he
tries to embrace you, say "no way" with a wicked glint in
your eye. Or, if you're usually "too tired", drag him to bed
and ravish him like a sex kitten.

· Demand his tongue, lips and hands on your hotspots. Or if
you usually call the shots, turn into his sex slave.

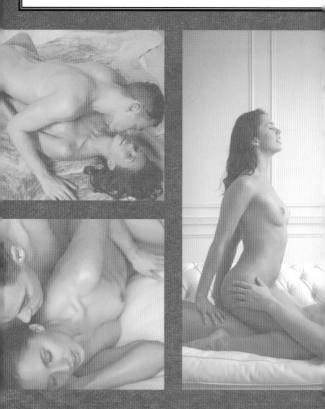

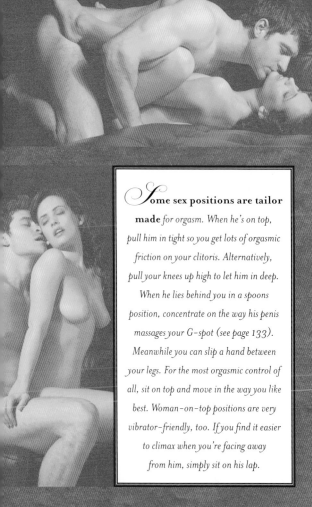

Some **sex positions are tailor made** *for orgasm. When he's on top, pull him in tight so you get lots of orgasmic friction on your clitoris. Alternatively, pull your knees up high to let him in deep. When he lies behind you in a spoons position, concentrate on the way his penis massages your G-spot (see page 133). Meanwhile you can slip a hand between your legs. For the most orgasmic control of all, sit on top and move in the way you like best. Woman-on-top positions are very vibrator-friendly, too. If you find it easier to climax when you're facing away from him, simply sit on his lap.*

The Secret Grip

*H*ave you ever tried lying still and making love using muscle power alone? All you need are strong pelvic floor ("PC") muscles and a willing man. And, as I've discovered, strong PC muscles bring other sexual benefits, too: you'll have more powerful orgasms and your vagina and G-spot will become super-sensitive.

TEST YOUR MUSCLE POWER

*I*magine you want to stop yourself from peeing – tense those muscles. To strengthen your PC muscles, lie on your back on the bed/floor with your knees bent. Imagine that your lover is inside you and you're trying to grip his penis hard. Squeeze your vaginal muscles tight (but keep your abdominal muscles and the rest of your body relaxed). Hold the squeeze for at least four seconds, then relax completely. Repeat this five times in a row and try to do it three times a day. During sex, use your PC muscles to grip him for as long as you can and use a combination of fast and slow squeezes.

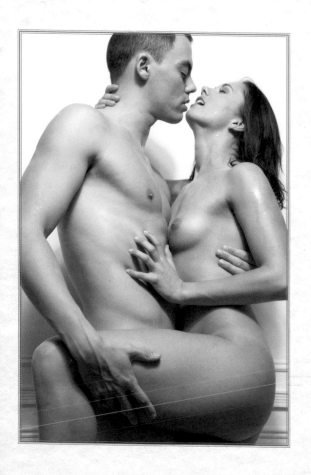

Naughty

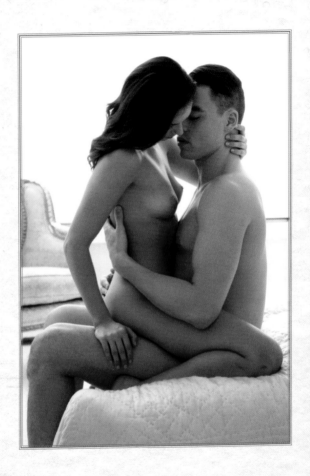

Naughty

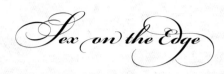

Sex on the Edge

I discovered a new place to have sex – somewhere that was not only super-erotic, but orgasm-friendly for both of us. I took my lover by the hand and led him to the bed. He looked perplexed until I positioned myself on the edge of the mattress and beckoned him over.

SPLIT-LEVEL SEX

Try these suggestions:

· You get on all fours on the edge of the bed and he enters you from a standing position. You get all the naughty thrills of the doggie position but without the hard friction on your knees. Plus, you can stimulate your clitoris while he thrusts.

· You stand on the floor and lean forward so your forearms are resting on the bed. He stands behind you and enters.

· You lie on your back on the bed. Your bum is near the edge and your feet are flat on the floor. Then he picks up your legs and puts them wherever he wants.

· He sits on the edge of the bed and you sit on his lap.

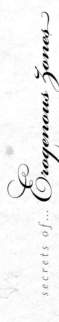

secrets of... *Erogenous Zones*

NAUGHTY NECKING

When my lover uses this technique, it always make me swoon with pleasure. He comes up behind me, twists my hair in his hands and lifts it up to expose the nape of my neck. He kisses this amazingly sensual spot, then uses his tongue and teeth to lick, nibble and graze the back of my neck and shoulders. Mmmm ...

WRIST KISS

Ask him to softly press his lips on the inside of your wrist and keep them there. Now get him to pull away and plant a row of really soft kisses along your inner arm.

LIP LOVE

Men tend to concentrate on the clitoris during foreplay, but remind him that your labia are full of nerve endings, too. Ask him to tweak and stroke them for meltingly erotic pleasure.

GIVE EACH OTHER'S TOES A TREAT

Get him to hold your foot firmly and slip his lips over your big toe, then slowly slide it in and out of his mouth with plenty of tongue pressure. Now return the favour.

GO DOWN ON HIM

Lie between his legs as if you were giving him oral sex, but, instead, go lower. Nuzzle and kiss the area just behind his balls – his perineum. Inflame him by exploring this neglected area thoroughly with your tongue.

PAY HIM LIP SERVICE

Instead of kissing his lips, gently caress them with your fingers. Run the tip of your index finger around the outline of his lips, then slip your finger provocatively into his mouth. Again, he'll associate it with fellatio – a real turn-on.

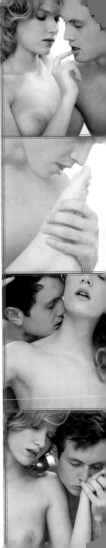

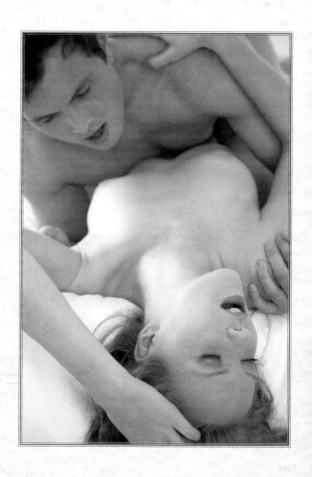

Naughty

Slowing Him Down

If your lover excels at the quickies but not the slow-burners, you'll be pleased to know there are some sexy and effective secrets for delaying his orgasm.

SLOWING-DOWN TECHNIQUES

- Full-body relaxation — as your partner ascends the arousal scale, you'll probably notice his breathing gets shallower and his body gets more tense and rigid. When he tells you he's getting as high as a seven or an eight, ask him to relax his body. Encourage him by stroking his belly, chest or shoulders and taking several deep, calm breaths in time with him. This should stop his arousal zooming up to a nine or a ten.
- Switching focus — instead of thinking about the sensations in his penis, he switches his focus to parts of his body where the sensations feel good, but not orgasmic.
- When he's super-skilled at pinpointing the high points of his arousal and getting himself back down to, say, a five, a six or a seven, he won't even need you to stop stimulating him.

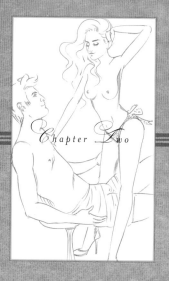

Chapter Two

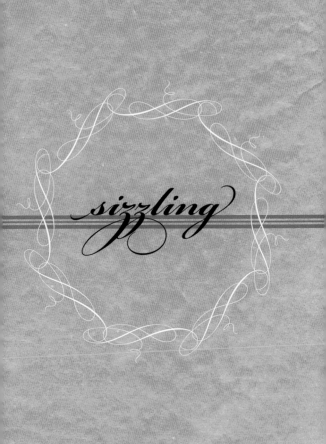

sizzling

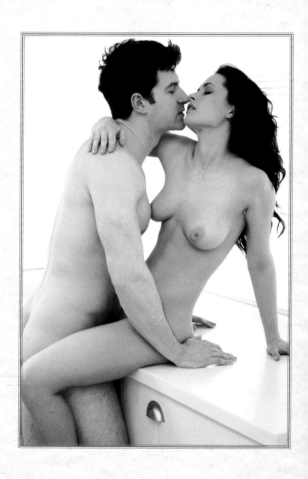

Sizzling

The Art of the Quickie

Whenever I want to feel desirable, wicked and wanton I suggest a quickie. It is a great way of reviving the heady, lust-driven early days of your relationship and the naughty glow lingers for hours afterwards.

QUICKIE SECRETS

Here are three facts that might challenge what you think about quickies:

- You don't have to be in a red-hot relationship to have a quickie. In fact, you can even use quickies as a form of sex therapy if your lovemaking has taken a nosedive.
- Quickies can be romantic. Especially if you gaze into each other's eyes all the way through. And especially if you call each other later on to say: "I love you — that was really fantastic."
- You don't have to be turned on before you embark on a quickie. It often works to throw yourself into the action and trust your body to respond.

WORK TO A DEADLINE

*T*he best quickies are when you've got only a tiny window of opportunity. Try this: initiate sex when you've got a set-in-stone deadline. For example: a train you have to catch or someone arriving for dinner. One of my most thrilling quickies was in a train compartment. We could hear the ticket collector coming toward us shouting "tickets please". As well as focusing your body and mind on the task, a deadline makes you more excited than usual. Try this five-minute sex schedule: one minute of kissing and foreplay; three minutes of sex; and one minute to make yourself presentable again.

QUICK STARTS

A request for quickie sex will almost always put a smile on your lover's face.

- Whisper a filthy proposition in his ear.
- Push him against a wall and kiss him hard.
- Guide his hand under your dress/skirt.
- Go up to him at a party, fix him with a wicked look then drag him to the bathroom.
  - Stop him at the door and say for him to pass, you have to have your way with him.

48

SEXY MIDDLES

There's no time for niceties in quickie sex. If you're going to go down on him — or him on you — pull his penis out of his trousers and go for it. And as soon as he's hard and you're wet, take the minimum of clothes off (ideally, just your panties) and slip him inside you.

Choose the position that allows you both to reach a fast climax. He'll need to thrust freely and you may need hand-room to stimulate your clitoris. Standing rear-entry positions are good — just find a nearby desk, table or other surface to lean on. Alternatively, sit on a counter, table or car bonnet and pull him between your legs.

I tend to throw in more kinkiness than I usually would. It adds to the sense of wildness and can get you to the peak quicker. Talk dirty to speed things up.

HAPPY ENDINGS

Try not to speak to each other after you've had quickie sex — add to the excitement and naughtiness by just communicating with eye contact and naughty grins. If one of you has to leave, try to say goodbye to each other with a passionate kiss and no words.

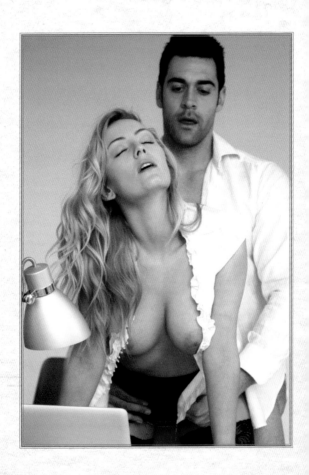

Sizzling

Beyond the Bedroom

$\mathcal{W}$ant to know a secret that will instantly transform your sex life? Give up having sex in bed. For me, moving sex out of the bedroom has always added a frisson of naughtiness — and, often, a thrilling challenge, forcing me and my lover into some sexy teamwork. It's helped me to discover the raunchy joys of sex positions that just don't work on a mattress — standing doggie, for example, and given me some unforgettable sexy memories.

IS THIS SEAT TAKEN?

$\mathcal{C}$hair sex is one of the first joys you'll discover when you get frisky away from the bed. It feels wickedly impromptu, and it means you can assume delicious erotic control by straddling him and bouncing up and down. And he gets passionately pumped as he sits back and admires the view. If you want to try something kinky with your lover, get him to sit on a dining room chair, then tie his wrists and ankles to the chair legs. Now you're free to give him a blowjob or sit on his lap, whatever takes your fancy.

IN THE DRIVING SEAT

*H*aving sex in a car is an exciting homage to adolescent lust. Play romantic or raunchy music — anything that matches your mood. And always park somewhere completely legal, with no one around for miles. Have sex on the car instead of in it. Use the car bonnet in the same way you'd use a kitchen counter (read on!). For extra naughtiness, lie back on the bonnet and ask him to give you oral first.

IF YOU CAN'T STAND THE HEAT ...

*S*ex in the kitchen offers the fantastic benefit of wicked and wanton counter sex. I love the drama of knocking the dishes aside in urgent lust, then brazenly jumping onto the counter, leaning back and pulling him in deep. Men love this position because it gives them the ability to thrust freely while standing with no weight to support. Try this for achingly deep and sensual penetration: instead of letting your legs hang off the counter, put your heels on the edge and pull your knees into your chest. Now guide him into you.

GOING WILD IN THE GARDEN

*S*lipping outside for an erotic tryst in the garden can make sex feel both risqué and romantic. If your garden is heavily overlooked, wait until it's completely dark, take cover in a pop-up tent or try my "invisibility" tips (see page 104).

Have sex on a tree – look for low boughs you can sit on, sturdy trunks to lean on; or branches to hang off.

HOT 'N' WET

*G*etting jiggy in the shower is sensual bliss – picture jets of water bouncing off you, steam caressing your bodies, fingers gliding over wet curves. My favourite position for shower sex is standing doggie – you lean forward and press your hands against the wall; he penetrates from behind. Your G-spot receives an orgasmic massage, and he gets a titillating view of your bum.

Try stepping out of the shower for your climax scene. My best bathroom poses are bending over and hanging on to the sink (great for eye contact in the mirror) and him sitting on the closed toilet lid with me straddling him.

Sizzling

Sex at Work ...

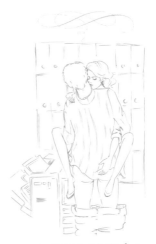

I'VE HAD SEX IN SOME UNUSUAL PLACES, but never at work. I've always been curious to find out what the appeal of this particular venue is. Is it just the thrill of being caught out? Is it the fact that you're doing something far more exciting than your usual work? These are some of my favourite explanations:

"I'm the keyholder to my office and sometimes my boyfriend comes to meet me at work when everyone else has gone home. We've often had standing-up sex with me leaning over the edge of my desk. I like it because it feels so wrong! I've spent all day being good, polite and professional, and sex in the office is a reversal of all that. We found that high-tech office chairs are great for having sex — the ones where you can adjust the height and tilt really far back."

"I met my boyfriend at work and we had to keep our relationship a secret in case it was frowned upon by our colleagues. But we took every opportunity to be naughty when we were out of sight — I gave him oral sex in the stationery cupboard and we had sex in the toilet and even on the fire escape. I'm sure other people do the same — offices are melting pots of sexual tension."

"My boyfriend and I had sex on my boss's desk. It was amazing, and it felt particularly naughty because I had a bit of a crush on my boss at the time."

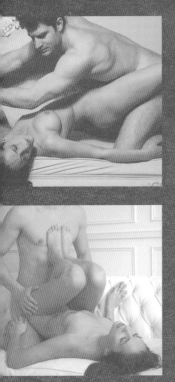

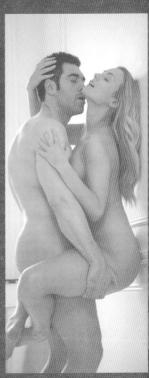

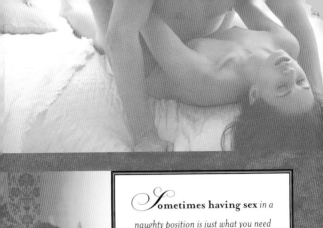

$\mathcal{S}$ometimes **having sex** in a
naughty position is just what you need
to take you over the edge and increase your
chances of having an out-of-this world
orgasm. Having sex while
standing up always feels thrilling,
but you can make it even more X-rated
by doing it pressed up against a wall
(especially if he picks you up).
You can make man-on-top positions
extra erotic by opening your legs
in a wide "V", by pushing your hips
up in the air or by pulling your knees
into your breasts.

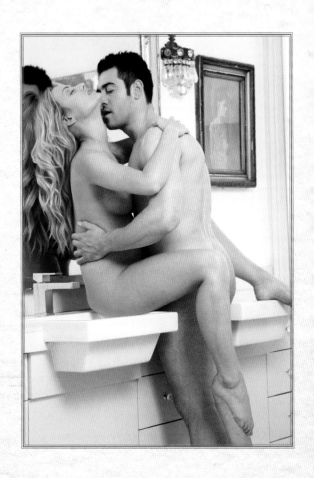

Sizzling

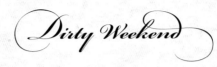

Dirty Weekend

Dirty weekends can invigorate your sex life – the erotic afterglow stays with you for days, plus you'll feel fantastically naughty, and deeply connected with your lover. Perhaps the best part is that you've got rid of everyday distractions – so you can shed your inhibitions and try those sexy acts you've fantasized about.

BEFORE YOU GO

I try to take as little as possible with me when we go away for a dirty weekend – I tend to stick to only sensual or sexy items. Include any of these in your weekend bag: thongs, stockings, basque, blindfold, massage oil, feathers, condoms, silk bathrobe, sexy dress, erotic novel, perfume, candles, iPod loaded with sexy music. Men love surprises that cater specifically to their sexual tastes. For example, if blowjobs are your lover's thing, he will be really delighted if you pull out some edible lube from your suitcase and offer to apply it for him.

DAY I

*W*hen you arrive go straight to bed. Plan to get frisky in various places: up against the door, in the shower, in an armchair, in front of a window or a mirror, and on the balcony or in the pool.

Treat everything that happens from now on as foreplay – even if you have a shower, make it slow, luxurious and steeped in eroticism. Discover each other's naked bodies beneath or on top of the sheets. Taste each other's lips. Tour his body with your tongue. Give each other a long full-body massage and lingering kisses. When you couldn't be any more aroused, take it in turns to ask each other for sexual favours. When it's your turn, describe what you want in lascivious detail. Make this erotic turn-taking the theme for the whole day. Include it in everything you do, even the things that aren't explicitly sexual, for example, "I'd like you to feed me dinner". Wait until night-time to have explosive sex that leaves you totally exhausted in each other's arms.

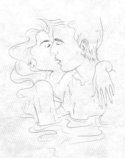

Today try things you've never tried before. Create some red-hot memories. Here are some ideas to inspire you:

- Render him completely helpless by blindfolding him in a dark room and binding his wrists and ankles. Put earphones into his ears and play him some sexy music. Now "torture" him with sexual treats.

- Explore the fetish world of "WAM" (wet and messy). Cover the floor with sheets or towels and wrestle, wriggle and writhe together while covered in a slick, wet, slippery substance such as oil, cream, body lotion or honey.

- Try body painting — it's a sexy way to become intimate with your lover's body and him with yours.

- Take advantage of the fact that you're in a hotel room — dress up as a kinky chambermaid and treat him to a teasing roleplay. Address him only as "sir".

- Take it in turns to give each other a genital massage for at least 20 minutes. When it's your turn to massage him, use long, sweeping, exploratory strokes that don't lead him straight to orgasm.

- Try disappearing from the hotel room for long enough to make your lover concerned, then send him a text telling him to come to the hotel bar. Throw yourselves into a strangers-meeting-for-the-first-time roleplay.

Sizzling

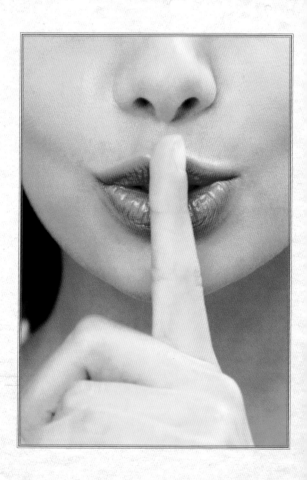

Sizzling

What's Your Pleasure?

*D*id you know that women can have different types of orgasm? These are clitoral orgasms, blended orgasms and uterine orgasms. Once I learned about the possibilities, I had a great time experimenting to see which kinds of touch triggered which kinds of orgasm.

THE EXPLOSION — CLITORAL ORGASMS

*A*s the name suggests, this orgasm comes from stimulating the clitoris. Most women climax this way by rubbing the clitoris with one hand. At the peak moment you experience intensely pleasurable feelings centred in your clitoris (I think of it as a "clitoral explosion") and the vaginal muscles contract rhythmically. My favourite "alternative" way of having a clitoral orgasm is to direct a stream of water from the showerhead onto my clitoris as I masturbate. Wonderful!

Another way, rather than attempting the in and out thrusts of intercourse, is to have internal, Tantric-style sex that relies on vaginal squeezes and penile flexes. Even if it doesn't give you an orgasm, you'll feel incredibly naughty, and you can carry on at home later. If you can't resist up and down movements, make them slow and infrequent. Or have quickie sex in minutes (see pages 47–9).

A THRILLING COMBINATION — BLENDED ORGASMS

In my experience, blended orgasms feel less "sharp" or localized than clitoral ones, but feel more intense emotionally and take a bit longer to "come down" from. Blended orgasms happen when the clitoris and vagina, most specifically the G-spot (see page 133), are stimulated at the same time. They're sometimes called "G-spot orgasms". The few times I've had one, I've felt quite a different sensation, because both the vaginal and uterine muscles contract.

For a blended orgasm, try any of these techniques:

· Stroke your clitoris while your lover massages your G-spot by hand.

· Use a rabbit vibrator, which is designed to stimulate the clitoris and the vagina/G-spot at the same time.

· Have intercourse — the head of your lover's penis thrusts against your G-spot, while the base of his penis rubs your clitoris (or use your fingers on your clitoris).

You'll probably find that a blended orgasm feels more subtle. Read these three descriptions:

"It feels softer and slower — like my whole body is involved."

"Deep, widening and pulsating. It touches something deep in me."

"A sense of deep release, but without the sudden piercing pleasure in my clitoris."

To find out if you can ejaculate, spend a while rubbing your clitoris and G-spot, and follow my tips (see page 110).

THE BIG WHAMMY — UTERINE ORGASMS

The uterine orgasm is considered to be the most rare but most deeply satisfying orgasm. It comes about as a result of deep rapid thrusts (from a penis, hand or sex toy) that jostle the cervix high up in the vagina. During the orgasm the uterus contracts rhythmically sending deep ripples of pleasure through the body. A uterine orgasm is thought to be the most intensely emotional (sometimes described as "earth-shattering"). Expect to cry, laugh or scream! And you'll probably need time to come down from the high. To explore uterine orgasms, you'll need to stimulate your A-spot —it's high up on the front wall of the vagina.

Try squatting, or drawing your knees up to your chest while you lie on your back. They're not the most dignified positions but they really help your lover to discover your A-spot.

USE THE STOP-START TECHNIQUE

Each time you feel yourself getting close to orgasm, stop all stimulation, and take some long, deep, belly breaths. This will take you back to a plateau of arousal — now work your way back up to a state of high excitement. Repeat this stop—start process until you can't bear it any longer — then surrender to an intense orgasm.

RELAX, RELAX, RELAX

Consciously relax your PC muscles (see page 36) so you're not holding even the tiniest bit of tension in your genitals (think of the level of relaxation you need to pee). I've found that having sex in this profound state of relaxation always gives me incredible orgasms.

GIVE HIM THE LOOK OF LOVE
To achieve the maximum in soul-baring intensity, try to hold your lover's gaze for the duration of your (and his) orgasm.

FOCUS ON THE DETAILS
The tingling in your thighs and genitals, and the melting sensation in your belly. When I do this, the small sensations come together in a big, glorious crescendo.

BE SELFISH (OR SELFLESS)
Sometimes I like dedicating an entire sex session to my orgasm or to his orgasm, but not to both. This way we each get all the attention and focus we need.

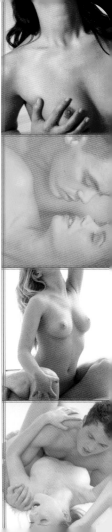

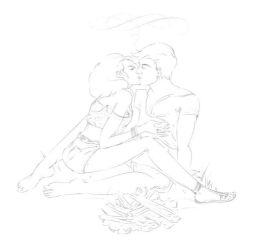

I LOVE STORIES in which people find themselves witnessing an erotic act — and getting helplessly turned on by it. These are two of my favourites:

"My partner and I saw something really erotic at a festival. We were sitting by our camp fire when we saw a couple go into their nearby tent and switch on a torch. The torchlight had the amazing effect not just of illuminating the tent but of creating big theatrical silhouettes of the couple's bodies. As they started undressing we looked discreetly away. But we couldn't resist looking back. The couple were sitting up kissing and stroking. It was like watching an erotic shadow play — we couldn't tear ourselves away. My partner snuggled up behind me and started to kiss my neck and caress my breasts. It was delicious. I'm ashamed to say that we spied on the couple all the way through to their climax scene. Then we had sex ourselves. It was wickedly exciting."

"As a film-maker I was once asked to document a Tantric sex workshop. I went along with a professional mindset — my job was to be the impartial observer and film what was in front of me. In practice, it wasn't so easy. The participants started off with a massage and some sensual dancing. But by the end of the workshop I found myself filming eight naked people all writhing on the floor. All I wanted to do was join in. I'm proud to say I maintained my professional front. But afterwards I rushed home, full of sexual tension, and pounced on my lover."

Amazing Oral

The ultimate erotic act ... that's how many men think of fellatio. It's hot, wet, tightly targeted stimulation and sublimely intimate, not to mention sexy. My top tip: learn how to enjoy yourself while you're doing it.

GIVE WITH PLEASURE

As you head south to give your lover oral pleasure, think about the tremendous sexual power you're about to wield. See it as an act of love, acceptance and trust.

To give an extra-special blowjob caress his testicles, perineum or anus as you go, and vary your mouth moves. Swirl your tongue around his glans on your upward strokes; flick your tongue all over his shaft and testicles; lick him as if you're trying to sculpt an ice-cream; and use your hand and mouth in tandem. My lover is really turned on when I surprise him with a blowjob in a semi-public place. I once went down on him while he was doing his accounts. It was quite clear which activity he enjoyed most.

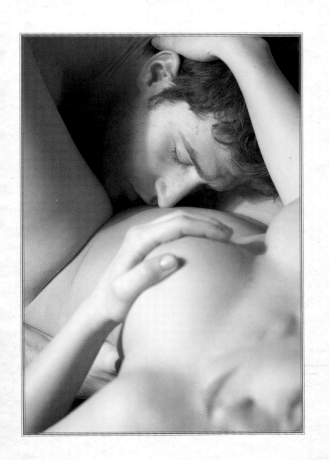

Sizzling

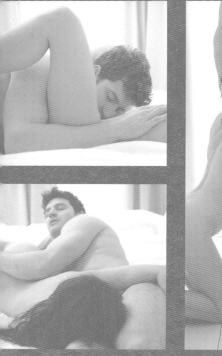

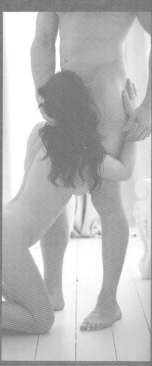

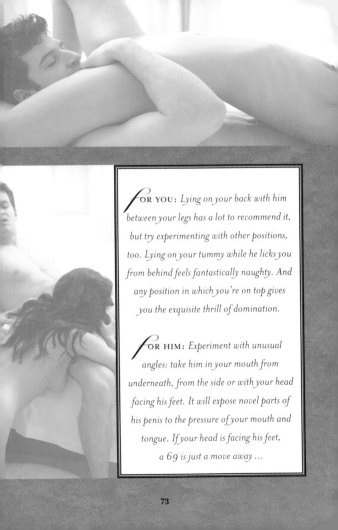

FOR YOU: Lying on your back with him between your legs has a lot to recommend it, but try experimenting with other positions, too. Lying on your tummy while he licks you from behind feels fantastically naughty. And any position in which you're on top gives you the exquisite thrill of domination.

FOR HIM: Experiment with unusual angles: take him in your mouth from underneath, from the side or with your head facing his feet. It will expose novel parts of his penis to the pressure of your mouth and tongue. If your head is facing his feet, a 69 is just a move away …

SIP CHAMPAGNE

Put the sizzle into sex with a little alcohol. Too much can hamper sexual response. My advice is to treat it as a romantic luxury and drink it in moderation. Great things have happened when I've begun the evening with a glass of champagne.

TAKE HIM TO AN OYSTER BAR

Casanova is said to have eaten 50 oysters for breakfast daily. Oysters aside, any food that has an erotic look helps put you in the mood for passion. I love figs, pomegranates, peaches and cherries for their voluptuous naughtiness. Nibbling fruit/licking juice from my lover's naked body is super-sexy.

GO HERBAL

Many herbs are touted as aphrodisiacs but few actually make the grade. One exception is rhodiola. It's said to not only enhance libido, but to improve

physical performance, boost energy
levels and combat fatigue – perfect
for long, lustful nights.

USE LAVENDER OIL

Smell has a massively potent effect on
desire. Strangely, researchers found
that the smell of lavender and pumpkin
pie are most stimulating to men.
Try them!

SNIFF HIM

Try having no-holds-barred, sweaty
sex. Perspiration secreted during sexual
arousal contains pheromones that can
act as powerful aphrodisiacs. Prepare
for a wild night.

SPICE THINGS UP

Hot and fragrant spices are reputed to
inflame the libido. Ginger is said to
be "the food world's Viagra". Pepper,
cardamom and chillies are also said
to boost sexual desire.

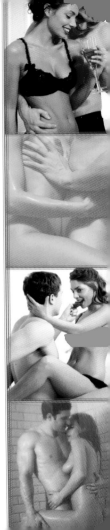

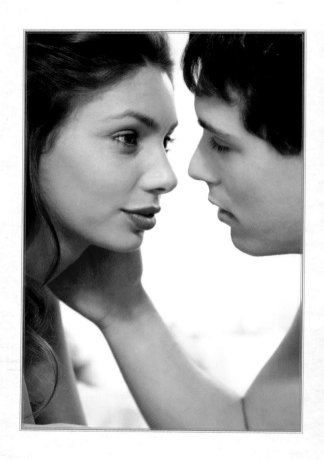

Sizzling

Tantric Pleasure

$\mathcal{T}$antra encourages you to have slow, sensual sex. You bond slowly with your lover until you reach a blissful peak of physical and emotional intimacy. Even then, you can simply bask in pleasure with no pressure to orgasm. It's said that Tantra "puts the soul back into sex". Rather than thinking about what you're doing, you're just following your body. One of the things I love about Tantra is that it shows my lover a more feminine way of having sex. He becomes more tender, and I'm more able to lie back and relish the sensations of sex.

CREATE A LOVE NEST

$\mathcal{I}$ learnt from Tantra to keep my bedroom clutter-free and more conducive to lovemaking. I make sure there's no dirty laundry, electronic gadgets and other distractions, so that I can relax as soon as I step through the door. I use candles, throws, cushions and exotic-smelling incense, such as cinnamon or sandalwood.

LOSE YOURSELF IN DANCE

Play your favourite music (preferably something rhythmic, trance-like or hypnotic) and, if the mood takes you, get up and dance. You might feel silly (I felt self-conscious at first), but free-form dance is a great way of losing yourself and becoming fully present in your body.

ENJOY SENSUAL TOUCH

Take turns to give each other a slow, sensual massage. Unlike an erotic massage in which you'd aim to build up genital arousal, you're going to include your lover's genitals in the massage, but without singling them out for any special attention.

YAB–YUM POSITION

When you're both in a cloud of sensual pleasure, get into the classic Tantric position known as "yab yum". If you like this position, you can go on to have sex in it later. Ask your lover to sit cross-legged on the floor, then sit in his lap so that you're facing him with your legs wrapped around his body and your feet behind his back. Once you're in this close Tantric cuddle, hold each other tight and enjoy the sensation of warmth being exchanged between your bodies.

When you're sitting comfortably, start to synchronize your breathing. Inhale and exhale softly through your nose, making your breaths increasingly long, smooth and flowing. When your breath is in a perfect seductive rhythm with your partner's, imagine that any boundaries or obstacles between you are melting away. Let the flow of your combined breath transport you to a place of peaceful love where there's nothing to do, say or think. All you have to do is sit quietly in each other's presence. If you are becoming aroused, embrace the feelings and allow them to intensify, but don't feel that you've got to speed things up, initiate sex or stimulate your partner.

SOUL GAZING

As you sit in the yab-yum position, hold each other's gaze. Don't stare each other out — just receive the gaze in relaxed intimacy. Let your desire build — imagine arousal swirling up from your genitals into your belly. When you're ready, put your hand on your lover's genitals and guide his hand to yours. Caress each other slowly. When or if you have sex, make it close and intimate with small rocking movements that gradually take you higher.

Sizzling

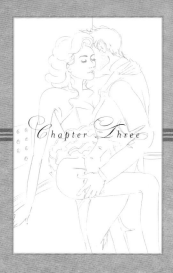

Chapter Three

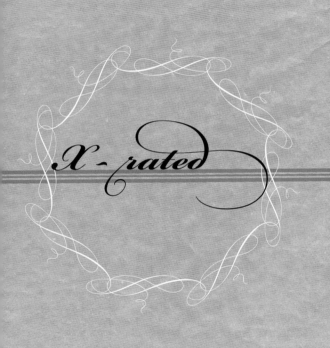

X-rated

LOVE YOUR BODY AND GET NAKED

The simple truth is that men love the sight and feel of a naked woman, plus they love a woman who's unhibited enough to "go for it" and really enjoy having sex. Hurrying to hide under the covers won't encourage him to ravish you. Joyously offering your body — however imperfect — will.

LOOK MESSY AND WILD

Forget about your hair and make-up. Let yourself get dishevelled in bed. Tousled hair and flushed cheeks are hot and will turn him on.

MOAN AND GROAN FOR HIM

Don't rush to impress your lover with your sexual repertoire — sometimes just responding to his lovemaking techniques will be enough. An ecstatic moan can go a long way to making him happy. And if he brings you to orgasm, he'll be as thrilled as you are.

MAKE EYE CONTACT

Whenever you have a peak lust moment, meet your lover's gaze and hold it for a few seconds. Sharing pleasure through eye contact is explosively intense.

FIND HIS TRIGGERS

Whether it's thigh-nibbling, hair-pulling or ear-nuzzling, most of us have personal triggers that turn us on. If you make the effort to discover your lover's special turn-ons, you'll be able to turn him to putty and pay him the compliment of truly understanding him sexually.

TRY THE "INNOCENT" LOOK

Men like outrageously naughty lingerie, but some find plain white undies an incredible turn-on — maybe it's the innocent and virginal overtones. Try slipping into bed in a pair of simple white cotton briefs and a vest.

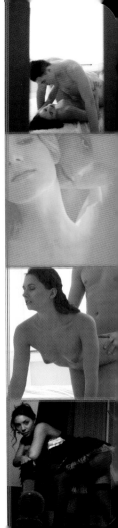

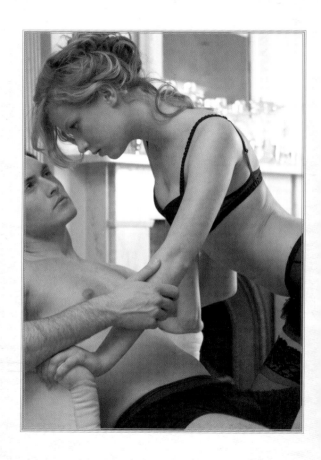

X-rated

Unleash Your Exhibitionist

If you don't count yourself as a natural exhibitionist,
and want to develop your "look-at-me" skills, read on ...

LET GO ...

- Before I put on a show for my lover, I find it helps to get to know myself in the mirror. Try out a variety of naked poses and moves — you'll quickly become comfortable with your own image. You'll also learn to judge what you like doing and what you don't and, importantly for your self-confidence, what looks good.
- Wander round the house wearing something provocative — whatever makes you feel confident and sexy.
- Undress in front of your partner when you're getting ready for bed — relish the feeling of his eyes upon you.
- Inject sexiness into the way you sit, stand and walk. Visualize a woman you consider sexy and copy her moves.
- Try sexual positions that put the spotlight on you — he lies flat on his back and you hop astride. Bask in the attention.

Sexy Stripping

If you want to wield sexual power and send him cross-eyed with lust, there are few better erotic treats than a striptease. And if, like me, you don't have a perfect body, don't worry: your lover will be so busy delighting in the show, he won't be casting a critical eye over you.

HOT TIPS

Remember:

- Don't wrestle with tops that need to be pulled over your head; wear garments that can be sexily unzipped or unbuttoned.
- Wear a skirt or dress that can be shimmied down your body.
- Stockings are a must — smooth them slowly down your thighs.
- Remember the mirror is your best friend — it'll teach you how to be stunning.
- Revel in your sexual power. Show your lover that you're having fun by holding his gaze; tease him by getting close then moving away; stick your bum out and wiggle it; lean over him so he has a great close-up view of your cleavage.

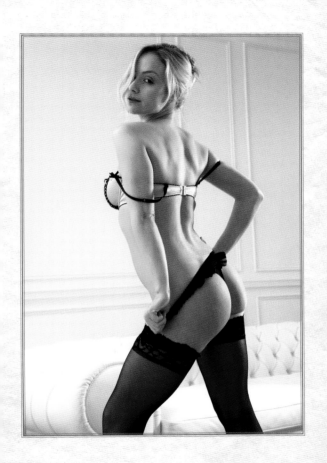

X-rated

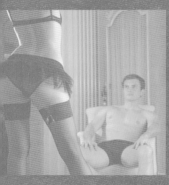

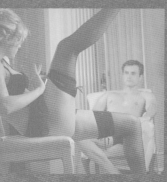

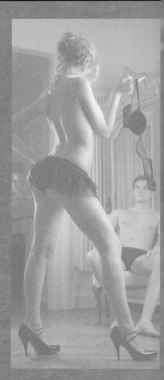

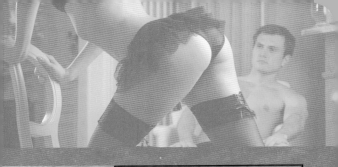

*B*efore you begin, *let yourself
be inspired by the classic moves shown
here. Make sure that your lover is sitting
comfortably, switch the music on and begin
your performance. Remember:
use the chair to show off your body.
Lean against the back and stick your
bum out, then sit down and raise a leg.
Trace the outline of your thighs as you
push your stockings off. Tease your lover by
making your moves slow and tantalizing.
When you take your bra off, dangle it
provocatively before dropping it.
End your striptease facing him so
he can feast his eyes upon you.*

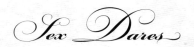

Sex Dares

*If you haven't left your sexual comfort zone recently,
try playing sex dares. I've always found it a great way to
shake up my sex life, and I love thinking up naughty
things I can do with my lover.*

PLAYING THE GAME

Get two pieces of paper. Each write down a list of sex
dares or "sexcapades" in the categories: "Easy", "Full-on" and
"I couldn't possibly do that … or could I?" For example:

• Easy: have a Brazilian wax; let him give me oral sex outdoors;
act out a scene from an erotic movie.

• Full-on: have webcam sex; describe then demonstrate how
I like to pleasure myself; play kinky doctor and nurse …

• I couldn't possibly do that … or could I: reveal a really kinky
fantasy; make a sex film; have anal sex; be a dominatrix.

Allocate your dares to three piles according to their category.
On a weekly dare night, pluck a slip of paper from the easy
pile. You can work up to the "I couldn't possibly …" dares.

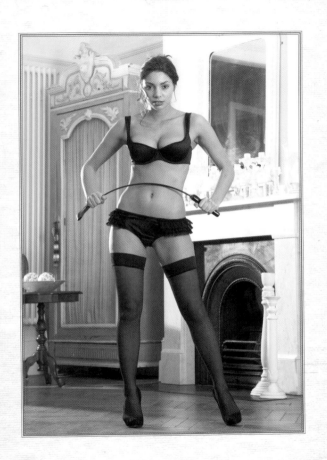

X-rated

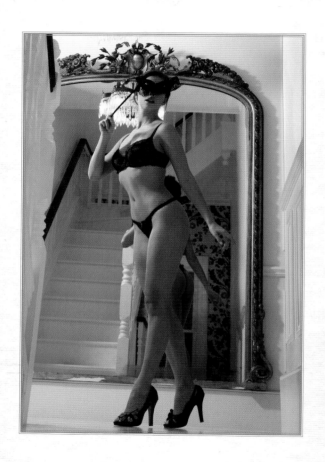

X-rated

Raunchy Roleplay

There's something amazingly erotic about pretending to be someone else, plus it means I can do things that ordinarily would make me blush. Try roleplaying when you're in the mood for a sexual adventure. Start by asking yourself who you want to become; and how far you'll go to bring your role to life. Roleplaying can be light-hearted and frivolous or used to explore your deepest, darkest desires. On the light-hearted side, you could act out a fantasy between two strangers at a masked ball. On the darker side, you could play master and slave games. How far you go is up to you.

BEFORE YOU BEGIN

Most roleplaying games involve a difference in power — that's what gives roleplay its special frisson. So, if you're new to roleplaying, sit down with your lover and answer the questions that are on the following page (do this separately, then compare your answers):

- Do you fantasize about being in charge and having complete sexual control?
- If you're in charge, would you be kind and giving, or bossy and strict?
- Do you fantasize about being helpless in bed?
- If you'd like to be helpless, do you like the idea of being overpowered or "taken"?
- Do you want to play different roles depending on your mood — sometimes dominant, sometimes submissive?

Now talk to your lover about how your fantasies could fit together. Does one of you want submission and the other dominance, or do you both crave either one? How do you feel about overpowering each other? Women who have lots of responsibility, pressure and commitment in their life tell me they find it liberating to be helplessly dominated during sex — to finally let go and let someone else be boss. But if you're shy and retiring, you may find it exciting to let your powerful and commanding side out to play.

WHO WILL YOU BE TONIGHT?

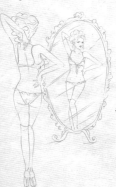

- *Voyeur and exhibitionist* — you're in your bedroom, taking your clothes off, caressing yourself. When you're naked and turned on, you start masturbating.

Outside the bedroom door is a stranger who's been spying on you. He's extremely excited — what happens next?

· Sex therapist and client: you're visiting a sex therapist and it's his job to make you come using different methods. For professional reasons he can't indulge his own lust. Will you force him to misbehave?

· Boss and employee: you're the boss and working late with your employee. You start asking him to do increasingly intimate jobs from taking your shoes off, to massaging your feet, to undressing. He must carry out the jobs willingly and ask for nothing. When he's granted all your sexual requests, you have to decide whether to reward him.

· Escort and client: you've sought the services of a male escort for one night only. He's happy to do anything. Before you take your clothes off and get started, he questions you about your favourite sexual acts.

· Slave and master: you've been naughty and need discipline. Your master's job is to deliver erotic "punishment", such as spanking. If you're good, he'll reward you with oral sex or other sexual treats.

· Artist and model: the artist insists that you pose naked for him. You enjoy the eroticism of lying back knowing that every curve of your body is being observed and enjoyed.

Dressing Up ...

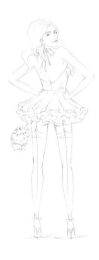

**I'M A RECENT CONVERT TO
CORSETS.** I love the way
they mould my body into a
perfect curvy shape and push
my breasts up to make me
look super-voluptuous. They
change the way I act in bed,
too — more brazen, more
confident and more in
charge. And, as I discovered,
I'm not alone in my love of
sexy costumes. Here are three
confessions from women who
always like dressing up before
going to bed ...

"My boyfriend bought me a chambermaid
outfit. It's brilliant and so much fun!
He finds it almost impossible to take his

eyes off me when I put it on. I do the classic chambermaid routine of dropping something, then slowly bending over in front of him so he can see my crotch outlined by my panties. I tie him up with a feather boa, too. It's great because normally I'm pretty reserved and dressing up gives me more sexual confidence."

"I went to a fancy dress party with an erotic theme and dressed up in this amazing catsuit. It was black latex. It was so skin-tight it left nothing to the imagination. I'm happy to say that evening restored all my sexual confidence – I could just see the lust in people's eyes."

"It doesn't sound very risqué, but my favourite sexy outfit is a satin Japanese kimono that just about covers my bum. Underneath I wear a gorgeous pair of crotchless lace briefs and nothing else. It makes me feel incredibly feminine. My biggest turn on is watching my lover's face as I stand by the bed and slide the kimono over my shoulders. I deliberately pause for a few seconds before revealing my breasts, then I let the kimono drop to the floor as I slowly slip into bed."

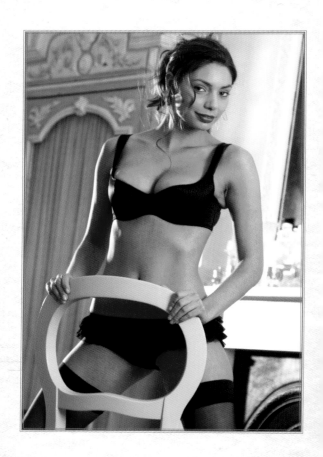

X-rated

Become an Erotic Dancer

Dancing for your lover is an amazing experience
— as well as taking him to a peak of excitement,
you'll get drunk on erotic power. You don't have
to be a great dancer — you just have to discover your
inner diva and embrace her with open arms.

THE MOVES

Start by positioning your chair facing your partner. Now
stand a couple of steps behind it, close your eyes and immerse
yourself in the opening notes of the music …

1 Stand with your legs apart and hold onto the back of your
chair. Lean forward to show lots of cleavage. Swirl your hips in
large slow circles or figures of eight. Bend your knees in time
with your moves. Keep your back straight and your head up.

2 Strut sexily from the back of the chair to the front — take
high steps and place each foot exactly in front of the other
foot, swaying your hips provocatively as you go. Leave one
hand on the back of the chair as you strut and, to sit down,

place your feet wide apart, keep your back straight and sway your hips from side to side until your bum meets the seat.

3 Sit on the chair with your thighs pressed together. Slip your fingers between the tops of your thighs and then slide them down your legs "forcing" them apart until they're in a provocative, wide-open "V" position.

4 With your legs still wide apart and your hands resting on the top of your thighs, move your hips in circles. Slide your hands up your thighs and over the front of your body.

5 Swivel on your chair by 45 degrees so you're sitting side on. Keep your legs together. Grip the edge of the seat behind you. Thrust your breasts forward and arch your back. Now rock backward and forward on your seat. Push your breasts out as far as you can.

6 Move to the edge of the seat. Keep rocking but make it incredibly slow. On a backward rock, lean back more than usual and raise one straight leg seductively in the air. If you can, point your toe to the ceiling. Lower your leg. On the next backward rock raise the other leg. Keep doing this.

7 Now swing one leg over the back of the chair so you're straddling the seat with your back to your lover. Grip the back of the chair with your hands and do the slow spin-a-hoop move you did in step 4. Again, get your chest and shoulders in on the act. Tip: keep changing the direction of your hip circles.

8 Stop circling your hips and slowly get up so you're in a standing straddle. Take hold of the back of the seat and pull it out from between your legs. Turn the chair round so you can grip the back. Take a few steps back until you're bending over almost at right angles. Now move your bum in circles or figures of eight (as you did in step 1). Push your bum as high in the air as you can.

9 Slowly stand up and turn to face your lover. Strut sexily toward him, then straddle him so that your breasts are positioned tantalizingly close to his face.

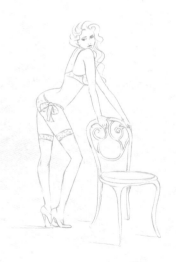

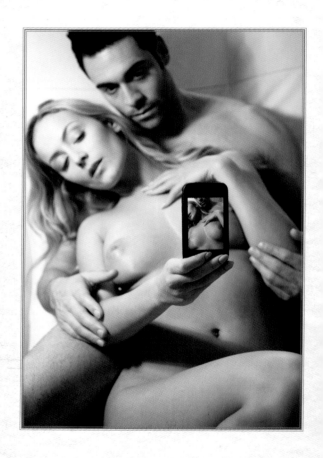

X-rated

Shoot Your Own Erotica

A naughty film is fun to make and thrilling to watch back later. "Home videos" are my favourite adult viewing – they kick-start sex when I watch them with my lover. Before you start, promise that anything you create will only be seen by each other. Or, if it makes you more comfortable, watch the footage once, then delete it.

THE **XXX** ACTION

When you're in the throes of passion, try to remember at least some of these secrets of on-camera sex:

- Do a bit of everything: he goes down on you, you go down on him, then when you have sex, keep switching positions.
- Include sex toys to keep the action varied.
- Make sure you both climax – it's exciting to watch back.
- Make your thrusts, grinds and wriggles big and dramatic.
- Connect your camera to a television so you can see what you're filming. Seeing the action unfold sends your arousal levels sky-high.

Sex in Public Places

If you've ever been aroused by the idea of having sex around other people, you're not alone. The idea of doing something naughty in public has always turned me on. But, as I've discovered, it's important to know how not to get caught in the act.

THE ART OF INVISIBILITY

*D*ress for the occasion. This means easily liftable skirts/ dresses (and no panties) and easy-access flies. A boyfriend once advised me to dress smartly because if you look formal, people are more likely to give you the benefit of the doubt.

Position is everything—arrange your bodies in a way that's as ambiguous as possible. I once had a fantastic afternoon in a park while curled up in a spoons position under a blanket.

Rather than attempting the in and out thrusts of intercourse, have internal, Tantric-style sex that relies on vaginal squeezes. If you can't resist up and down movements, make them slow and infrequent.

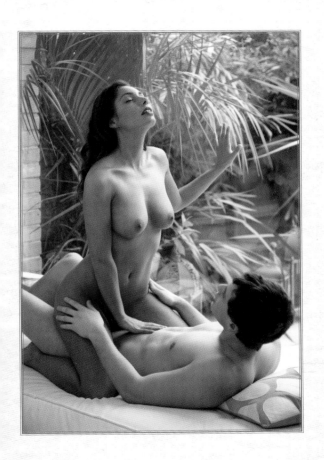

X-rated

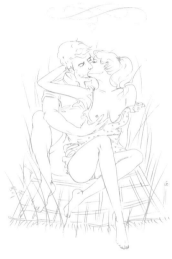

SHORTLY AFTER WE FIRST STARTED GOING OUT, my lover took me on a very sexy picnic in the countryside. Instead of sandwiches, he packed cream, honey, strawberries and champagne. I knew things were going to become fun when he started drizzling the honey on me. But for me, the highlight was just being naked outdoors with the sun on my body and the grass tickling my skin. I've always found something very sexy about being close to nature. As I went on to discover, I'm not alone:

"I went on a walking holiday with my boyfriend and we found ourselves on a remote beach sheltered by a high cliff. There was no-one around for miles and my boyfriend, who's a keen photographer, suggested that I strip off so he could take pictures of me. I found it so sensual to lie naked in the sand or pose on rocks. Both of us got incredibly turned on and ended up having wild sex in the sea."

"Forests do it for me. I love the idea of sneaking off into the woods for secret sex, which I used to do with my first boyfriend. I don't know whether it's the possibility of getting lost, being discovered or the naughtiness of being taken up against a tree. I find it very exciting."

"We climbed a mountain once on holiday. We were so exhilarated by getting to the top, we made love standing behind a rock. It was one of the best sexual highs I've ever had!"

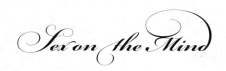

Sex on the Mind

I've discovered the more naughty thoughts I have, the more sexual attention I get from my lover, partly because I initiate sex more, and partly because I'm already raring to go when he's in the mood. When I start thinking sexy, I become more sensual. I wear perfume to bed, give my lover sensual massages and make food to share in bed.

THINK SEXY

*M*ake sex your new hobby:

- Plan a "sex date", then lose yourself in erotic anticipation before the event. Imagine the things you'll do, your seduction techniques and the positions you'll try.
- Reminisce about a favourite erotic encounter or dream up a sexual fantasy. (I often revisit a holiday I had in Greece). Share your thoughts with your lover by text, email or letter.
- Keep erotic reading beside the bed.
- Make sex a conversation piece with female friends — ask if they've ever tried a particular position/toy/technique.

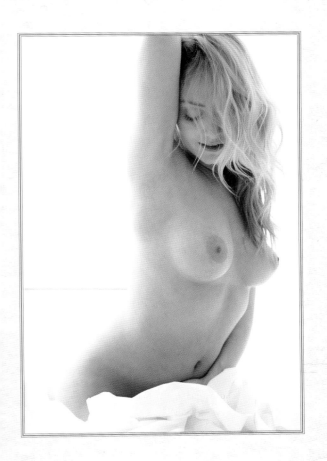

X-rated

BELIEVE IT'S POSSIBLE
Explore your body with an "anything-could-happen" mindset.

DOUBLE THE PLEASURE
Use your index finger to gently stroke or tickle your clitoris while your other hand massages your G-spot (see page 133). If this sounds like too much multi-tasking, ask your lover to help.

GO G-SPOTTING
Ejaculation happens during G-spot stimulation, so you'll need a very hands-on relationship with yours. If you can't find your G-spot with your fingers, invest in a G-spotter (vibrator with a curved or bulbous end). If you can find your G-spot with your fingers, rub it firmly in small circular movements. Continue and soon your G-spot will get larger and change in texture. Now just keep going ...

LIE BACK AND RELAX

Aim for really deep relaxation that allows you to shed your inhibitions and abandon yourself to pure eroticism. The biggest block to ejaculating is fear of letting go. It's advisable to empty your bladder completely as this helps you to relax, and if you do ejaculate, you can be sure it's not urine.

PUSH!

When you're close to coming, remove your fingers and push down/let go as if you're trying to pee. This will make you ejaculate if you're going to. If it doesn't work the first time, keep alternating G-spot stimulation with pushing down.

BE STRONG

If you've got strong pelvic floor muscles, you're more likely to ejaculate. Do the PC workout on page 36, starting now.

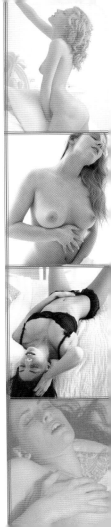

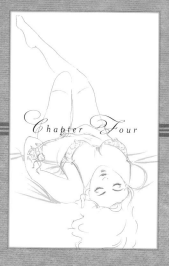

Chapter Four

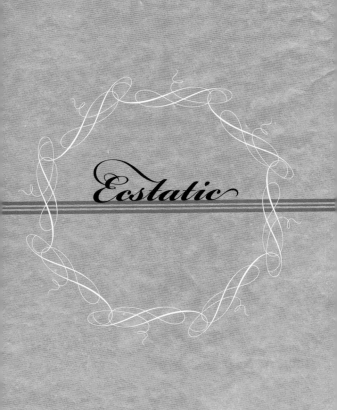

Ecstatic

Get What You Want

*I*t's incredibly titillating for my lover when I tell him what I want. He loves to get some guidance from me. Asking for what you want means you get the right stimulation exactly where, when and how you need it.

KNOW WHAT TO SAY ...

*D*rench your requests with praise, encouragement and compliments. For example, if he hears that you love a particular technique — and you just want more of it, or you just want it softer or harder, he'll be delighted. Criticism is a no-no in the bedroom — it's a massive passion killer and can result in less sex rather than better sex. Make your requests precise. Leave him with no uncertainty. For example, say, "I'd like you to put your fingers inside me while you give me oral sex." Give him a sexy guided tour of your body or touch yourself in front of him. You could make it into a roleplaying game. Pretend you're virgins and have to rely solely on each other to learn about the opposite sex.

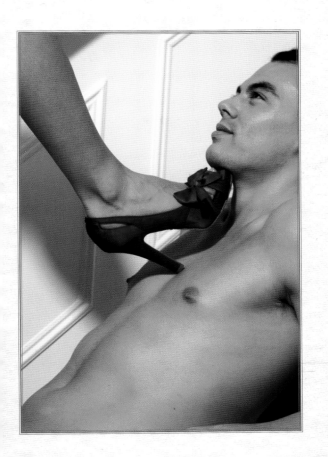

Ecstatic

PRACTICE MAKES PERFECT

Discover what gives you most pleasure and then show your lover. Masturbate in an alternative position, such as standing up or sitting. Or use a new technique. Try thrusting against a pillow or using your "wrong" hand. Using various techniques is a great way to become more orgasmic.

DOUBLE STIMULATION

Try massaging the clitoral head (the bud you can see) with one hand while moving your fingers or a vibrator in your vagina with the other hand. The friction will indirectly stimulate the rest of the clitoris (the invisible bit hidden inside your body), which gets stiff and erect when you're turned on.

READ ...

Sex for One: The Joy of Self-Loving by Betty Dodson, who's famous for her "genital show-and-tell" group masturbation sessions.

GO ELECTRIC

Use a vibrator. A close friend of
mine who had never had an orgasm
confided: "Once I found out what a
vibrator orgasm was like, I learned how
to get there with my hand."

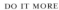

DO IT MORE

Research shows masturbation increases
self-esteem, sexual confidence and
satisfaction levels. Women who
masturbate have more orgasms with a
partner. Masturbation also makes you
more comfortable with your body,
relieves stress and menstrual cramps,
and even helps you get to sleep. What
are you waiting for?

TAKE A DETOUR

Turn yourself on by stroking and
tweaking your inner labia before
you zone in on your clitoris. These
sensitive lips are often neglected, but
they're rich in nerve endings and can
take you to new ecstatic heights.

117

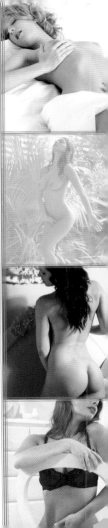

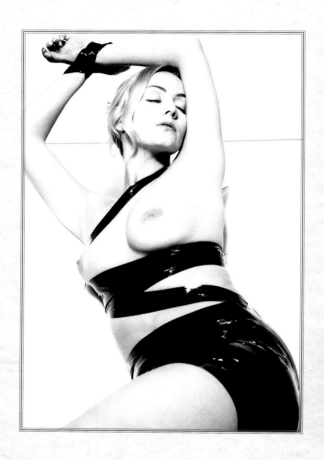

Ecstatic

Sexy Bondage Techniques

Tying up your lover is a great way to take control. The reason I enjoy it: if he can't move, he can't call the shots, and that's perfect because it means I'm free to demand sexual favours or tease him until he's completely weak with lust. I've noticed that men are reluctant to admit they like the vulnerability of being tied up. Yet once they're bound to the bed they find it incredibly erotic. Take the lead – tell him you're doing it for your own pleasure rather than his.

GATHER YOUR PROPS

Most people think of ropes and handcuffs when they think of bondage, but unless you want to engage in serious kinkiness, these are some of the friendlier options for making your lover into a sexy captive:

- Silk scarves – these are great because they can serve a dual purpose. After you've wafted them seductively over your lover's body, in particular his penis, balls and belly, you can use them to tie his ankles and wrists to the bed. Just don't tie silk scarves too tight (and keep a pair of scissors handy in case the knots are difficult to undo).

- Bondage tape — it might sound daunting, but bondage tape is one of the simplest and safest types of restraint (great for beginners). The first time you use it, wrap it around your captive's ankles or wrists.
- Velcro cuffs — You can find fur-lined cuffs with quick-release Velcro fastenings in any online sex shop. They're quick and easy to slap on him when he's been naughty and they won't cut off his blood supply.
- Spank ties — these bendy toys are perfect for novices. They're lengths of flexible metal coated in comfortably soft rubber. As well as being easy to use, they're surprisingly versatile. They can be used to give your lover a naughty spank before tying him up.

GETTING INTO A BIND

The most popular position for being tied up is lying spread-eagled on the bed. It's a bondage cliché, but it's got a lot to recommend it: it leaves the captive's genitals exposed, which provides intense erotic vulnerability, and easy access to hotspots; and because the captive's arms are secured, there's no choice but to surrender.

When tying your lover's hands together, instead of binding his wrists with the palms face to face, tell him to cross his wrists in front of his body, then wrap a long, skinny scarf around them in a criss-cross fashion. This not only looks sexier, it also allows him to put his arms behind his head while you have your wicked way with him. Let him do the same to you.

RULES OF ENGAGEMENT

*E*ven if you're only doing some light dabbling in the world of bondage, follow these safety guidelines:

- Agree a codeword that means "stop, I've had enough". Always choose something other than the word "stop" because shouting this is often part of the fun and so can lead to misunderstandings.
- Don't tie your lover up and leave him on his own.
- Don't tie anything around the neck, and don't cut off circulation — you should always be able to slide one or two fingers between your lover's skin and the restraint.

Power Games ...

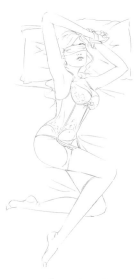

I ONCE ASKED A FRIEND why she was so into power games with her boyfriend. She looked at me directly and said: "for the orgasms". According to her there's something about being submissive that takes arousal to new heights. And she said that with extreme arousal comes extreme and highly pleasurable orgasm.

She told me, "I find that there's something incredibly liberating about being submissive. He simply tells me what to do and I do it. Sometimes he makes his authority clear by physically restraining me. Other times, he'll threaten to spank me if I don't "behave". Sometimes he just uses the tone of his voice and body language. There's something thrilling about completely surrendering to someone. Being submissive makes all my normal hang-ups disappear. If he tells me to crawl across the bed on all fours, I'll happily do it. There's no thought involved — I don't think "Should I be doing this?" I just do it. I get completely immersed in the moment and I absolutely love it.

Another great benefit of submission is that it makes me the centre of attention. People assume that if you're submissive, you're the less important partner. In fact, you're constantly in the spotlight because you're always being observed and told what to do. So being submissive makes me feel as if I'm the star of the show, but without feeling like an attention-seeking show-off. I also know that my lover is incredibly turned on by the games we play — and arousal is infectious. If I think he's getting a huge dose of pleasure, it has a knock-on effect on me. We drive each other to peaks of lust that feel addictive."

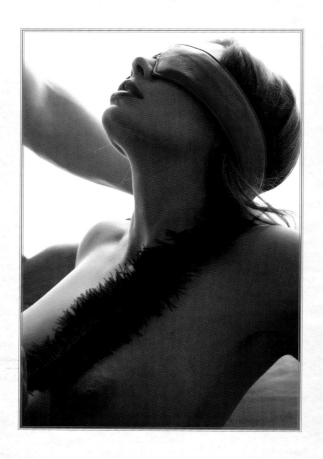

Ecstatic

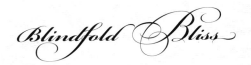

Blindfold Bliss

With a blindfold, you can enter the sexy world of surprise, sensuality and submission. Think of blindfolding as the extremely mild end of dominance and submission games.

SURPRISE, SENSUALITY AND SUBMISSION

- **Surprise**: You only know what's happening when your lover's body touches yours. As soon as you break contact, what will come next? Will he kiss you? Go down on you?
- **Sensuality**: Your other senses become sharper. You can lose yourself in the sounds, smells, tastes and tactile sensations of sex. Depriving your lover of his sight can feel liberating — you're free to look at him and marvel at his sexiness. And any inhibitions about your body vanish.
- **Submission**: Your lover has the power to tease, delight or torment. Yes, you can just rip off the blindfold in a second — but part of the fun of blindfolding is surrendering to your lover and being open to whatever happens.

Ecstatic Orgasms

One of the best ways to improve orgasms is to stop having them. I think of it as an orgasm diet. You don't have to give up sexual intimacy — the opposite, in fact. The whole idea of the orgasm diet is that you go back to the basics of intimacy and rediscover each other. You can space the four sessions over four nights, over a week, a fortnight or longer. If you enjoy one of the four sessions in particular, you can repeat it as many times as you like.

BEFORE YOU START

Make the following pact with your lover before you begin. Agree to:

· Wait until your fourth session before you have an orgasm.
· Only do things that feel pleasurable/fun/sensual. Stop if anything feels like hard work.
· Take away any performance pressure — there's no obligation for either of you to do anything.
· Relax during each session so that you're fully "present".

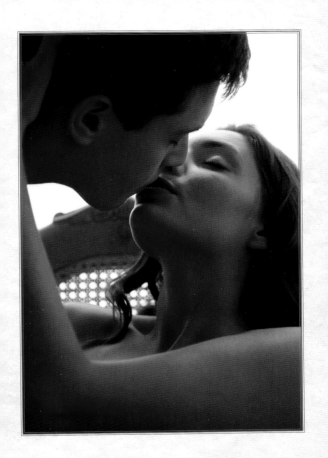

Ecstatic

SESSION ONE

*P*retend that you're learning to touch each other for the first time, with one important rule: you mustn't touch each other's genitals and nipples. Experiment with different types of touch: nibble each other's earlobes; have a steamy kissing session; kiss each other's toes; run your hands over each other's bum; lick a patch of skin and blow on it; caress each other with a silk scarf. Talk to each other — say what feels good, or just go "mmmmm …". Tease him by slipping your fingers under the waistband of his boxers. Let your hand linger for a few moments, then pull back.

SESSION TWO

*C*arry on exploring like you did last time, but include genitals and nipples. Let yourselves get turned on, but don't climax. Let arousal come and go — if he gets an erection, just include it in your explorations. If you want to give him oral sex, make it relaxed and pleasurable — for example, keep your mouth and tongue soft and find a comfortable position where he can stroke you at the same time. And get him to touch you in new ways, for example, his flat palm pressed against your vulva or a slow line traced from your clitoris to your vagina. If you want something in particular, ask.

SESSION THREE

This time when you're both aroused climb on top of him and slide his penis inside you. Rather than doing the usual in-out, grinding and rubbing movements of intercourse, just stay still or move very gently together. Savour the sensations, but don't let them build up to a peak. When you're sitting astride him, take his hands and pull him up to a sitting position. Wrap your arms around his body and give him a passionate kiss.

SESSION FOUR

This time you can both go as far as having an orgasm. Condense all the three previous steps into a single experience, building up gradually so that your route to climax is slow, sensual and meandering. If orgasm doesn't come naturally, don't make it into a goal – just let it happen (or not). Remember that your only aim is pleasure.

You may find you're so orgasm-hungry at the end of your diet, you'll be able to come in a completely different way from usual. Try experimenting. My lover managed to give me an orgasm using just his toe!

Ecstatic

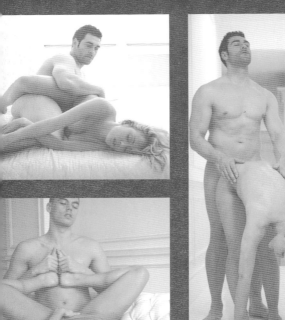

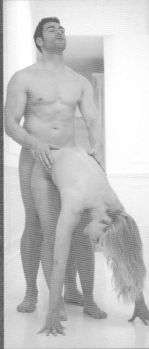

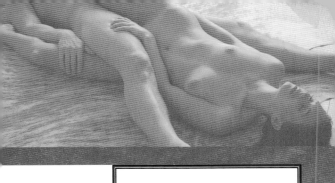

*𝒯***ry any of these** *sexual*
positions when you're in the mood
for more of a challenge.
Novel angles and positions can make
sex feel exciting and experimental.
You may even discover hotspots you
didn't know you and your lover had.
Even physically demanding postures,
such as bending forward to touch the floor,
are worth it for the psychological thrill.
Often, for him, it's all about the view.
If he can look down and gaze
at your bum or breasts,
he'll be in sexual heaven.

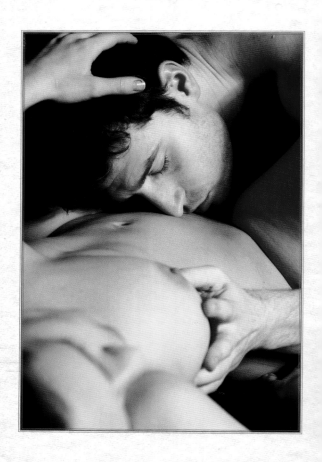

Ecstatic

G-spot Ecstasy

For explosive sex, guide your lover to
your G-spot. Most of us have heard of it,
but many women still find it elusive.

IN SEARCH OF THE G-SPOT

The G-spot is best explored when you're extremely aroused
– it swells when you're turned on and becomes easier to find.
Smooth your lubricated fingertips along the front wall of
your vagina and find an area that feels like a raised button.
Don't worry if you can't find this – some women experience
the G-spot as an area of general erotic sensitivity. Press and
massage the area and see what sensations you experience.

The first time a lover touched my G-spot I was sure I was
going to pee – this is completely natural and happens because
the G-spot is close to the urethra. Just see what happens.
Feelings could range from nothing to vaginal orgasm and
female ejaculation that give truly ecstatic pleasure.

Ecstatic Fantasies

A really sexy fantasy boosts my libido, gives me more intense orgasms, and makes me feel more sexually adventurous. And if I confess to something I'm embarrassed about and my lover goes along with it, I fall in love with him all over again. There's nothing wrong with borrowing or stealing other people's fantasies to get your creative (and other) juices flowing.

EROTIC REVELATIONS

Discuss how you can bring your fantasies to life or, if that's going too far, find some erotica that enacts your fantasy for you. Here's some confessions friends have shared with me:

"I'd love to have an orgasm when I'm out to dinner. I imagine my lover touching me under the table."

"I fantasize about being filmed while I'm masturbating."

"I've often imagined kissing another woman."

"I'd like my boyfriend to blindfold me and then be the boss."

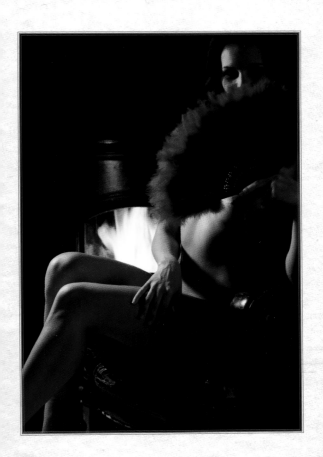

Ecstatic

INVENT A NEW SEX POSITION

Give your position an unlikely name. Discuss it with your lover innocently in front of friends: "Hey, do you fancy a chai latte when we get home?"

WOW HIM!

Buy a pubic hair stencil and wax your pubes into a heart or diamond shape. Or make your bare skin look gorgeous with stick-on crystals designed for this area.

TRY NAKED YOGA

Do a shoulderstand and ask him to give you oral sex. Prepare for a head rush.

HAVE ANIMAL SEX

He's a lion, you're a kitten, or vice versa.

69 WITH A TWIST

Get into a side-by-side 69 position.
Now instead of licking each other's
genitals, suck each other's toes.

HAVE FOOD SEX

Smother each other in anything sticky,
runny, creamy … When you can't
get any messier, press your bodies
together.

MAKE UP A SEX RULE

And he has to obey it for the night.
For example, no hands, only tongues;
or standing sex only.

PLAY SEXY HIDE AND SEEK

Each hiding place becomes the venue
for a naughty foreplay act.

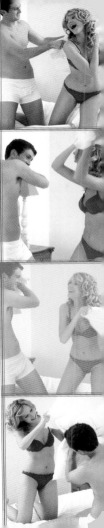

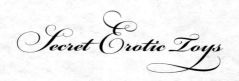

Secret Erotic Toys

A friend told me she improvised household objects as
sex toys. Afterwards I saw my electric toothbrush in a whole
new light! All it takes is a slightly kinky imagination.

IT'S PLAYTIME...

*H*ere's some suggestions...

- **Exercise ball** – try having sex on one. It's wobbly and
precarious, but great fun. Ask your love to straddle the ball,
then sit on his lap and bounce.
- **Oil drizzler** – fill an oil drizzler with sweet-smelling
coconut oil, then drizzle it over your lover's naked body.
- **Beanbags** – all sorts of sex positions feel fantastic on a
beanbag. The balls mould to the contours of your body.
- **Feather duster** – use it to tickle and polish your lover from
head to toe, then he can return the favour.
- **Clothes pegs** – if you want to make each other gasp, clothes
pegs are the perfect alternative to nipple clamps. Take turns
to put them on each other.

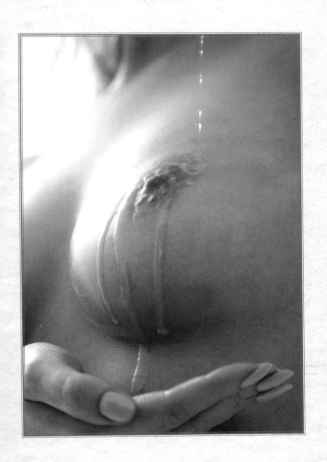

Ecstatic

BE AN ICE QUEEN
Get him to smooth an ice cube around your nipples or your labia, clitoris and vagina. Afterwards he can make you melt by dripping warm (but not hot) water directly onto your clitoris. Or he can lick you after taking a sip of hot tea.

GIVE HIM GLOVE LOVE
Blindfold him, lay him flat on his back and then stroke his erect penis with different types of gloves. Try a leather glove, a rubber glove, a woollen mitten or – my personal favourite – an elbow-length silk glove.

SPANK HIM
Softly caress his naked bum with your palm. Then give him two light taps followed by two hard spanks.

Then go back to soft caresses.
Always aim for the anal area —
never the tailbone — and keep
your hand slightly curved.

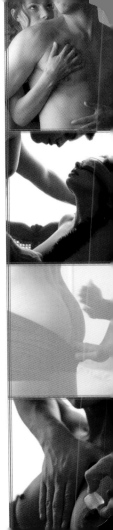

PLAY WITH DIFFERENT SENSATIONS
Use feathers to stroke, fingernails
to scratch or fingers to pinch.
Take it in turns to wear a blindfold
to heighten sensitivity.

GIVE HIM A HOT SURPRISE
Lay him down for a candlelit massage,
then pick up the candle and use it to
drip wax on him from the nape of
his neck to the cleft of his buttocks.
Rub the wax sensuously into his body.
Caution: use only "massage candles"
(the wax melts at a lower temperature
than normal candles).

Spanking ...

I HAD AN EXCITING EVENING of spanking recently.
Not the dress-up-as- a-schoolgirl type of spanking
– more a massage that turned naughty. I'd just
given my lover a back rub and was finishing off

with some strong hacking strokes. I noticed that everytime I hit his bum his moans got louder. So instead of using the sides of my hands, I started spanking him with the flats of my hands instead. He loved it.

I asked him to do it back to me and I found it not just erotic, but surprisingly sensual.

It seems that spanking is more popular than you might think, and with lots of people ...

"My partner sometimes spanks me during sex. It sends a shock wave of pleasure up my body and makes me gasp. I like the fact that I never know when he's going to do it."

"We discovered spanking when we were play-fighting. I was pretending to be really angry with him. I pulled his trousers off and began spanking him. I started getting really into it and couldn't stop! He got really turned on."

"I love the stinging sensation on my bum. It's not pain exactly. More like a hot, tingling feeling. I like it when he follows it up with a nice gentle massage, too."